300 Questions and Answers in Exotics and Wildlife for Veterinary Nurses

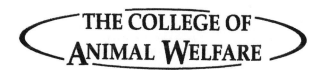

Senior commissioning editor: Mary Seager
Development editor: Caroline Savage
Production controller: Anthony Read
Desk editor: Angela Davies
Cover designer: Helen Brockway

300 Questions and Answers in Exotics and Wildlife for Veterinary Nurses

The College of Animal Welfare

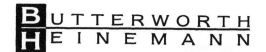

OXFORD AUCKLAND BOSTON
JOHANNESBURG MELBOURNE NEW DELHI

Butterworth-Heinemann
Linacre House, Jordan Hill, Oxford OX2 8DP
225 Wildwood Avenue, Woburn, MA 01801-2041
A division of Reed Educational and Professional Publishing Ltd

℞ A member of the Reed Elsevier plc group

First published 2001
Transferred to digital printing 2004
© The College of Animal Welfare 2001

British Library Cataloguing in Publication Data
300 questions and answers in exotics and wildlife for veterinary nurses
  1. Veterinary nursing – Problems, exercises, etc.
  I. College of Animal Welfare II. Three hundred questions and
answers in exotics and wildlife for veterinary nurses
636'.089'073076

ISBN 0 7506 4696 9

Typeset by Keyword Typesetting Services, Wallington

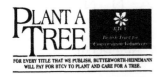

Contents

Acknowledgements

The College is most grateful for the help of the following colleagues in the preparation of this book:

C. Allan
B. Cooper
W. Fulcher
D. Gould
L. Tartaglia

Introduction

How the book is organized

This book of Exotic and Wildlife questions has been produced in response to further requests for more multiple choice questions. It contains 300 questions covering Exotics and Wildlife. After the questions is a list of correct answers.

How to use the book

Do your revision first, then select a range of question numbers at random. Do this without looking at the questions in advance. You should be able to complete and finish one multiple choice question per minute, allowing time for a thorough read of the question and the options before selecting the correct answer.

Questions

1) *What is the CORRECT name for the top half of a chelonian's shell?*

   a) Plastron
   b) Base
   c) Carapace
   d) Carabase

2) *What is the CORRECT term used to describe a snake's skull?*

   a) Brachycephalic
   b) Dolicocephalic
   c) Kinetic
   d) Fused

3) *In which part of the body would you find the 'spectacle'?*

   a) Ear
   b) Eye
   c) Nose
   d) Mouth

4) *What is the main excretory by-product of metabolism in all reptiles?*

   a) Urea
   b) Uric acid
   c) Nitric acid
   d) Ammonia

5) *Which reptile lacks a urinary bladder?*

   a) Chelonian
   b) Lizard
   c) Snake
   d) Tuatara

6) *From WHERE would you obtain a blood sample in the snake?*

   a) Jugular vein
   b) Dorsal tail vein
   c) Ventral coccygeal vein
   d) Cephalic vein

7) *How many digits are there on a tortoise's hind limb?*

   a) 3
   b) 4
   c) 5
   d) 2

8) *What is the function of the Jacobson's organ?*

   a) Balance organ
   b) Enhances taste/smell
   c) Detects heat
   d) Picks up vibrations

9) *What is the CORRECT term given to the most distal part of the digestive tract where waste is excreted?*

   a) Anus
   b) Cloaca
   c) Colon
   d) Ano-genital orifice

10) *Which class of reptile does the Mediterranean tortoise fall into?*

   a) Squamata
   b) Crocodylia
   c) Chelonia
   d) Tuatara

11) *Which essential vitamin does ultraviolet light provide for captive reptiles?*

   a) Vitamin B_1
   b) Vitamin C
   c) Vitamin D_3
   d) Vitamin E

12) *Which ONE of the following is NOT a classification of amphibians?*

   a) Limbless
   b) Tailed
   c) Tailless
   d) Newts

13) *Which ONE of the following terms BEST describes a reptile that lays an egg requiring incubation?*

   a) Oviparous
   b) Ovoviviparous
   c) Viviparous
   d) Voiloparous

14) *Which measurement is used to determine ideal weight for tortoises?*

   a) Janson's graph
   b) Jackson's ratio
   c) Newton's law
   d) Mayo's measurement

15) *Why do some reptiles need to hibernate?*

    a) Temperature too cold
    b) Not enough vegetation
    c) Need to sleep
    d) As a stimulus to breed

16) *How long before going into hibernation should food be withheld in the Mediterranean tortoise?*

    a) 1 week
    b) 3–4 days
    c) 2–3 weeks
    d) 2–3 months

17) *Which species rarely suffers from nutritional disorders?*

    a) Lizards
    b) Chelonia
    c) Snakes
    d) Tuatara

18) *Which ONE of the following have the greatest nutritional quality?*

    a) Mealworms
    b) Waxworms
    c) Locusts
    d) Crickets

19) *What is the MOST common disease found in captive reptiles?*

   a) Obesity
   b) Metabolic bone disease
   c) Kidney failure
   d) Iodine deficiency

20) *In which species is vitamin A deficiency common?*

   a) Tortoises
   b) Snakes
   c) Iguanas
   d) Red-eared terrapin

21) *What is the MAIN clinical sign of an animal suffering from vitamin A deficiency?*

   a) Anorexia
   b) Lethargy
   c) Swollen eyelids
   d) Excessive hiding

22) *In which species of snake is hypovitaminosis B_1 (thiamine deficiency) commonly seen?*

   a) Corn snake
   b) Royal python
   c) Garter snake
   d) Black mamba

23) *Thiamine deficiency in garter snakes may cause?*

   a) Skin lesions
   b) Rickets
   c) Lack of neuro-muscular coordination
   d) Anorexia

24) *Which definition BEST describes 'preferred body temperature'?*

   a) The highest temperature at which most reptiles can be kept
   b) The lowest temperature at which most reptiles can be kept
   c) The temperature at which a given species functions at its best
   d) A range of temperatures within the vivarium

25) *Which ONE of the following anaesthetic circuits is preferable for reptiles weighing under 5 kg?*

   a) Circle
   b) To and fro
   c) Ayres T-piece
   d) Magill

26) *Mediterranean tortoises are easily sexed once they reach maturity because males:*

   a) Have long claws on their front feet
   b) Are larger than the female
   c) Have a more concave shell
   d) Have more pronounced femoral pores

27) *In the tortoise, WHICH blood vessel is the MOST common site for taking a blood sample?*

   a) Jugular vein
   b) Cephalic vein
   c) Dorsal tail vein
   d) Ventral tail vein

28) *Which ONE of the following is the BEST method of handling a corn snake?*

   a) Restrain the head and let the rest of the body hang
   b) Restrain the head and support the weight of the rest of the body
   c) Lift the snake in the middle with two hands
   d) Place your hand into the vivarium and allow the snake to coil around your arm

29) *Which ONE of the following is the BEST method of transporting a snake to the surgery?*

   a) In a cardboard box with substrate
   b) In a cloth bag within a polystyrene styrofoam box
   c) In its vivarium
   d) Carry it in your arms

30) *Which method should be used to transport a red-eared terrapin?*

   a) A plastic box with a lid containing a damp towel
   b) A cardboard box with newspaper
   c) A bucket of water
   d) A plastic container with a small amount of water in it

31) *Which ONE of the following substrates should NEVER be used for reptiles?*

   a) Corn cob
   b) Gravel
   c) Cedar wood shavings
   d) Reptile carpet

32) *At which temperature should a green iguana be kept?*

   a) 20–25°C
   b) 26–30°C
   c) 30–35°C
   d) 35–40°C

33) *Which ONE of the following statements is INCORRECT?*

   a) Male iguanas have more pronounced femoral pores than the female
   b) Males are larger than females
   c) Males have larger dewlaps than the female
   d) Males are duller in colour than the female

34) *What is the average life expectancy of the iguana?*

a) 5–10 years
b) 10–12 years
c) 15–20 years
d) 20–25 years

35) *Which ONE of the following foods should be avoided in a tortoise's diet as it is low in vitamins and minerals?*

a) Mixed greens
b) Cucumber
c) Chickweed
d) Lettuce

36) *Which species usually only possesses one functional lung?*

a) Iguana
b) Red-eared terrapin
c) Snake
d) Tuatara

37) *Some snakes possess heat sensitive pits along their upper lip. What is their function?*

a) They do not have one
b) Pick up small rises in temperature to allow them to detect the presence of warm-blooded prey
c) It allows them to pick up vibrations from the ground
d) It is a way in which reptiles detect the time for hibernation

38) *What is the ideal environmental temperature range for the Mediterranean tortoise?*

a) 26–29°C
b) 25–40°C
c) 10–20°C
d) 40–45°C

39) *Which type of lighting system provides essential UVA/ UVB wavelengths for captive reptiles?*

a) Infrared lights
b) Hot rocks
c) Light bulbs
d) Fluorescent tubes

40) *Which ONE of the following would be the MOST appropriate diet for a 15 cm (6 inch) corn snake?*

   a) Mouse
   b) Rat
   c) Furry
   d) Pinky

41) *Which ONE of the following is NOT a clinical sign of nutritional osteodystrophy in the green iguana?*

   a) Dull/lethargic
   b) Anorexia
   c) Diarrhoea
   d) Muscle atrophy

42) *Which ONE of the following zoonotic diseases is the MOST common in captive reptiles?*

   a) Rabies
   b) Salmonella
   c) Psittacosis
   d) Giardia

43) *Which ONE of the following classifications does the cornsnake fall into?*

   a) Squamata
   b) Chelonia
   c) Crocodylia
   d) Anuria

44) *Which ONE of the following BEST describes the lifestyle of the green iguana?*

   a) Terrestrial
   b) Arboreal
   c) Aquatic
   d) Marine

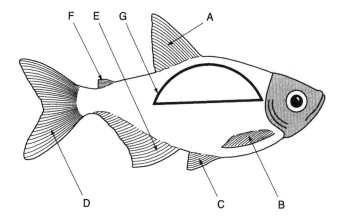

45) *With reference to the above diagram. What is the function of structure G?*

   a) Digestion
   b) Buoyancy
   c) Involved with gaseous exchange
   d) Storage organ

46) *What is the name of the fin labelled A?*

   a) Dorsal
   b) Pelvic
   c) Caudal
   d) Adipose

47) *What is the name of the fin labelled B?*

   a) Pelvic
   b) Adipose
   c) Pectoral
   d) Caudal

48) *What is the name of the fin labelled C?*

   a) Pectoral
   b) Caudal
   c) Pelvic
   d) Anal

49) *What is the name of the fin labelled D?*

   a) Pectoral
   b) Caudal
   c) Pelvic
   d) Anal

50) *What is the name of the fin labelled E?*

   a) Pectoral
   b) Caudal
   c) Pelvic
   d) Anal

51) *What is the name of the fin labelled F?*

   a) Pelvic
   b) Adipose
   c) Pectoral
   d) Caudal

52) *Which fins are paired?*

   a) Dorsal and caudal
   b) Anal and pectoral
   c) Dorsal and pelvic
   d) Pectoral and pelvic

53) *Which fins are used to keep the fish upright?*

   a) Dorsal and anal
   b) Pectoral and pelvic
   c) Caudal and adipose
   d) Anal and pectoral

54) *Which fins can be used to act as 'brakes' slowing the fish down?*

   a) Pectoral
   b) Dorsal
   c) Caudal
   d) Pelvic

55) *In fish, what is the function of the lateral line?*

a) To detect vibrations and currents
b) To detect chemical changes in the water
c) To aid the fishes sense of 'smell'
d) To detect the body heat of adjacent fish in shoaling species

56) *When introducing new fish into an aquarium, which one of the following is INCORRECT?*

a) The bag containing the new fish should be floated in the aquarium
b) Existing fish should be fed before releasing the new fish
c) Ideally new fish should be quarantined before introduction to an existing aquarium
d) The new fish should be floated in their bag for several days prior to release

57) *A tropical, freshwater aquarium containing many species of fish that live peacefully together is often called:*

a) A community tank
b) A group tank
c) A natural tank
d) A commune tank

58) *A fish that is swimming upside down and cannot right itself is most likely suffering from:*

   a) Gill flukes
   b) Dropsy
   c) Swim bladder disorder
   d) Anchor worm

59) *The condition known as white spot is caused by:*

   a) A virus
   b) A bacterial infection
   c) A fungal infection
   d) A parasite

60) *As a general rule of thumb, fish should be fed:*

   a) Once a week
   b) Ad libitum
   c) Small quantities 2–3 times per day
   d) A good handful once a month

61) *Which ONE of the following would not be a suitable live food for fish?*

   a) Leeches
   b) Daphnia
   c) Bloodworm
   d) Brine shrimp

62) *Which ONE of the following BEST describes the diet of an adult iguana?*

  a) Obligate carnivores
  b) Omnivorous, eating only a small quantity of meat
  c) Omnivorous, eating only a small quantity of vegetable matter
  d) Obligate herbivores

63) *Which ONE of the following species of reptile would be the MOST suitable as a pet for a 10-year-old child?*

  a) Burmese python
  b) Tokay gecko
  c) Leopard gecko
  d) Green iguana

64) *Which ONE of the following species of snake requires a diet of fish and worms?*

  a) Corn snake
  b) Milk snake
  c) Garter snake
  d) King snake

65) *Reptiles and amphibians can all be described as:*

  a) Ectothermic
  b) Endothermic
  c) Warm-blooded
  d) Ectodermic

66) *Many lizards shed their tails if startled or handled incorrectly. This process is known as:*
   a) Autonomy
   b) Autotomy
   c) Autolysis
   d) Sloughing

67) *The lower half of a chelonian's shell is called the:*
   a) Carabase
   b) Carapace
   c) Plastron
   d) Base

68) *The shields (or scutes) that run down the midline of the carapace are called the:*
   a) Pleural shields
   b) Nuchal shields
   c) Marginal shields
   d) Vertebral shields

69) *The shields of which shell can be used for individual identification?*
   a) Carabase
   b) Carapace
   c) Plastron
   d) Upper

70) *Which ONE of the following species of snake can be described as viviparous?*

a) Corn snake
b) Milk snake
c) Garter snake
d) King snake

71) *Red-eared terrapins are predominantly:*

a) Aquatic
b) Terrestrial
c) Arboreal
d) Marine

72) *Freezing whitebait prior to feeding to a garter snake may cause:*

a) Hypovitaminosis A
b) Hypovitaminosis B
c) Hypovitaminosis C
d) Hypovitaminosis D

73) *Which ONE of the following would be considered unsuitable as a pet for an adult with asthma?*

a) Corn snake
b) Leopard gecko
c) Cold water fish
d) Budgerigar

74) *Which ONE of the following species is classified as an invertebrate?*

   a) Snake
   b) Tarantula
   c) Bird
   d) Lizard

75) *Which muscle presents a suitable site for injection in the rabbit?*

   a) Triceps
   b) Pectoral
   c) Biceps femoris
   d) Quadriceps

76) *In rabbits, what is the COMMON term for the condition known as myiasis?*

   a) Fly strike
   b) Lameness
   c) Diarrhoea
   d) Weeping eyes

77) *Which ONE of the following zoonotic diseases can be transmitted by rodents?*

   a) Salmonellosis
   b) Psittacosis
   c) Giardiasis
   d) Ringworm

78) *Which ONE of the following zoonotic diseases can be transmitted by birds?*

   a) Scabies
   b) Salmonellosis
   c) Leptospirosis
   d) Rabies

79) *Leptospirosis occurs in which ONE of the following species?*

   a) Birds
   b) Foxes
   c) Ferrets
   d) Reptiles

80) *Leptospirosis is usually transmitted by contact with an infected animal's:*

   a) Faeces
   b) Urine
   c) Blood
   d) Vomit

81) *Which ONE of the following zoonotic diseases causes 'flu-like' symptoms in humans?*

   a) Salmonellosis
   b) Rabies
   c) Scabies
   d) Leptospirosis

82) *Which ONE of the following diseases is notifiable?*

   a) Viral haemorrhagic disease
   b) Myxomatosis
   c) Rabies
   d) Salmonellosis

83) *Which ONE of the following is NOT usually evident in small mammals in pain or discomfort?*

   a) Aggression
   b) Inactivity
   c) Anorexia
   d) Vocalization

84) *A tropical freshwater aquarium should IDEALLY be maintained at:*

   a) 14°C
   b) 20°C
   c) 25°C
   d) 35°C

85) *A goldfish can be described as what type of species?*

   a) Cold, freshwater
   b) Cold, marine
   c) Tropical, freshwater
   d) Tropical, marine

86) *Which ONE of the following species would be MOST suited to life in a pond?*

   a) Oranda
   b) Black moor
   c) Koi carp
   d) Neon tetra

87) *The amount of oxygen dissolved in the water of a tank depends upon:*

   a) The surface area of the tank
   b) The temperature of the water
   c) The presence of aeration devices
   d) All of the above

88) *Frogs and toads belong to which group?*

   a) Anura
   b) Caudata
   c) Apoda
   d) Chelonia

89) *Which ONE of the following groups is endothermic?*

   a) Chelonia
   b) Squamata
   c) Anura
   d) Mammalia

90) *Almost all adult amphibians are:*

   a) Herbivorous
   b) Omnivorous
   c) Carnivorous
   d) a or b

91) *The Axolotl is a larval stage of a species of:*

   a) Frog
   b) Toad
   c) Newt
   d) Salamander

92) *The major nitrogenous excretory product of fish is:*

   a) Urea
   b) Ammonia
   c) Nitrite
   d) Nitrate

93) *How many toes does a rabbit have on its forelimb?*

   a) 2
   b) 3
   c) 4
   d) 5

94) *What is the space between the incisors and molars of a rodent known as?*

   a) Open rooted
   b) Diastema
   c) Diallema
   d) Hard palate

95) *What are 'caecotrophs'?*

   a) Urinary deposits
   b) Soft pellets
   c) Dry pellets
   d) Diarrhoea

96) *How many toes does a guinea pig have on its forelimb?*

   a) 2
   b) 3
   c) 4
   d) 5

97) *Where is the scent gland located in gerbils?*

   a) Perineal area
   b) Above the tail
   c) Mid ventral abdomen
   d) Under the chin

98) *Which ONE of the following species of hamster has internal testes?*

   a) Syrian
   b) Chinese
   c) Russian
   d) Golden

99) *In gerbils, which type of food, if fed in excess, can cause skeletal abnormalities?*

   a) Cheese
   b) Raisins
   c) Sunflower seeds
   d) Maize

100) *What temperature is ideal for keeping hamsters?*

   a) 10–15°C
   b) 19–23°C
   c) 25–30°C
   d) Doesn't matter

101) *Which treat is LEAST appropriate to feed to a hamster?*

   a) Cheese
   b) Crisps
   c) Chocolate
   d) Mealworms

102) *Which vitamin is an essential part of a guinea pig's dietary requirement?*

a) Vitamin A
b) Vitamin C
c) Vitamin D_3
d) Vitamin E

103) *To which order do rabbits belong?*

a) Rodentia
b) Lagomorpha
c) Carnivora
d) Mustela

104) *At what age is a buck rabbit sexually mature?*

a) 4–5 months
b) 6–7 months
c) 10–12 months
d) 12–18 months

105) *At what age do the pelvic bones of the female guinea pig fuse?*

a) 3 months
b) 6 months
c) 8 months
d) 12 months

106) *Which ONE of the following species has precocial offspring?*

   a) Gerbil
   b) Hamster
   c) Rat
   d) Chinchilla

107) *Which ONE of the following guinea pig varieties BEST defines a single hair colour?*

   a) Agouti
   b) Marked
   c) Self
   d) Hooded

108) *Which ONE of the following coat types describes a smooth haired guinea pig?*

   a) Peruvian
   b) Abyssinian
   c) English/American/Bolivian
   d) Argentinian

109) *What is the gestation period of the rabbit?*

   a) 28–32 days
   b) 60–72 days
   c) 20–22 days
   d) 19–21 days

110) *What is the gestation period of the guinea pig?*

   a) 28–32 days
   b) 60–72 days
   c) 20–22 days
   d) 19–21 days

111) *What is the dental formula of the adult rabbit?*

   a) 1/1, 0/0, 3/2, 3/3
   b) 1/1, 0/0, 2/3, 3/3
   c) 2/1, 0/0, 3/2, 3/3
   d) 2/1, 0/0, 2/3, 3/3

112) *Which ONE of the following breeds of rabbit would be MOST suitable as a child's pet?*

   a) Dutch
   b) New Zealand White
   c) Angora
   d) Flemish giant

113) *Which ONE of the following rabbit breeds would have fur resembling velvet, lacking any guard hairs?*

   a) Angora
   b) Cashmere
   c) Dwarf lop
   d) Rex

114) *Which ONE of the following is NOT a breed of rabbit?*

a) Belgian Hare
b) Chinchilla
c) Angora
d) Chinese dwarf

115) *How would you confirm the sex of a female rabbit?*

a) By the fact that you could not feel any testicles in the scrotum
b) By the observation that it was smaller than others of a similar age
c) By examining the genital orifice and revealing a slit like opening
d) By examining the genital orifice and revealing a Y-shaped opening

116) *Against which ONE of the following diseases should pet rabbits be vaccinated in the UK?*

a) Distemper
b) Leptospirosis
c) Myxomatosis
d) All of the above

117) *Which ONE of the following should be a consideration regarding surgery in the rabbit?*

   a) Food should be withheld for 12 hours prior to anaesthesia
   b) Hyperthermia is a risk postoperatively
   c) Hypoglycaemia may develop postoperatively if the rabbit is not offered food soon after recovery
   d) All of the above

118) *Which ONE of the following statements is correct?*

   a) Rabbits are omnivores
   b) Ferrets are herbivores
   c) Rats are omnivores
   d) Mice are herbivores

119) *Which ONE of the following species has a furred tail?*

   a) Gerbil
   b) Rat
   c) Mouse
   d) Hamster

120) *The male of which species has two teats?*

   a) Guinea pig
   b) Rat
   c) Mouse
   d) Gerbil

121) *Which ONE of the following species does not have scent glands?*

a) Gerbil
b) Hamster (Syrian)
c) Rabbit
d) Rat

122) *What is the dental formula of the rat?*

a) 1/1, 0/0, 1/1, 3/3
b) 2/1, 0/0, 1/1, 3/3
c) 1/1, 0/0, 3/2, 3/3
d) 1/1, 0/0, 0/0, 3/3

123) *What is the term given to species that are active at dawn and dusk?*

a) Crepuscular
b) Diurnal
c) Noctural
d) Biurnal

124) *What is the gestation period of the Syrian hamster?*

a) 15–18 days
b) 28–32 days
c) 19–21 days
d) 60–72 days

125)   *Which species of hamster has a solitary lifestyle (except for breeding)?*

a) Syrian
b) Chinese
c) Russian
d) All of the above

126)   *Which ONE of the following materials would be unsuitable as bedding for a hamster?*

a) Shredded paper
b) Hay
c) Cotton wool
d) All of the above

127)   *Which ONE of the following terms BEST describes the diet of the Syrian hamster in the wild?*

a) Herbivorous
b) Omnivorous
c) Carnivorous
c) Frugivorous

128)   *Which ONE of the following species is prone to hibernation at temperatures below 5°C?*

a) Mouse
b) Rat
c) Gerbil
d) Hamster

129) *Which ONE of the following best describes the reproductive cycle of the Syrian hamster?*

   a) Seasonally polyoestrus
   b) Polyoestrus
   c) Monoestrus
   d) Dioestrus

130) *From where does the Chinchilla originate?*

   a) South America
   b) China
   c) Jamaica
   d) Syria

131) *What is the gestation period of the Chinchilla?*

   a) 18 days
   b) 28 days
   c) 62 days
   d) 111 days

132) *What is the average lifespan of the Chinchilla?*

   a) 1 year
   b) 4 years
   c) 10 years
   d) 25 years

133) *Which ONE of the following cages would be MOST suitable to house a single Chinchilla?*

   a) A wooden and mesh cage 2 m × 2 m × 1 m
   b) A plastic cage 2 m × 2 m × 1 m
   c) A metal, mesh cage 2 m × 2 m × 1 m
   d) Any of the above

134) *Chinchillas require daily access to a tray containing fine volcanic rock powder. The purpose of this is to:*

   a) Provide a way for the Chinchilla to clean its fur of grease and dirt
   b) Provide a vital dietary supplement
   c) Provide a medium for urination and defaecation
   d) Provide an opportunity for play behaviour

135) *What is the dental formula of an adult Chinchilla?*

   a) 1/1, 0/0, 0/0, 3/3
   b) 1/1/, 0/0, 1/1, 3/3
   c) 1/1, 0/0, 2/3, 3/3
   d) 2/1, 0/0, 2/3, 3/3

136) *Chinchillas are:*

   a) Herbivorous
   b) Carnivorous
   c) Omnivorous
   d) Frugivorous

137) *What is the average litter size of the Chinchilla?*

    a) 2
    b) 6
    c) 8
    d) 10

138) *What is the name given to the male guinea pig?*

    a) Buck
    b) Hob
    c) Cob
    d) Boar

139) *What is the alternative name for the guinea pig?*

    a) Cavy
    b) Cochon
    c) Small pig
    d) Guinean pig

140) *Which ONE of the following coat types describes the coat of a guinea pig that is in rosettes or swirls?*

    a) Peruvian
    b) Abyssinian
    c) English
    d) Argentinian

141) *Which ONE of the following coat types describes the coat of a long-haired guinea pig?*

a) Peruvian
b) Abyssinian
c) English
d) Argentinian

142) *Which ONE of the following BEST describes the reproductive cycle of the guinea pig?*

a) Seasonally polyoestrus
b) Polyoestrus
c) Monoestrus
d) Dioestrus

143) *Which ONE of the following statements is CORRECT?*

a) Guinea pigs are solitary animals and should be kept alone
b) Two female guinea pigs may not be kept together as they will fight
c) Two male guinea pigs may be kept together providing they are introduced at an early age
d) Males used for breeding will live happily with each other

144) *What is the dental formula of an adult guinea pig?*

    a) 1/1, 0/0, 0/0, 3/3

    b) 1/1, 0/0, 1/1, 3/3

    c) 1/1, 0/0, 2/3, 3/3

    d) 2/1, 0/0, 2/3, 3/3

145) *What is the term given to hypovitaminosis C?*

    a) Scurvy

    b) Coccidiosis

    c) Ringworm

    d) Enteritis

146) *What is the average litter size of the mouse?*

    a) 2

    b) 6

    c) 8

    d) 10

147) *What is the gestation period of the rat?*

    a) 20–22 days

    b) 28–32 days

    c) 18–20 days

    d) 60–72 days

148) *Which ONE of the following species would you expect to have the highest respiratory rate?*

   a) Rabbit
   b) Guinea pig
   c) Rat
   d) Mouse

149) *Which ONE of the following species has the longest average lifespan?*

   a) Rabbit
   b) Rat
   c) Hamster
   d) Mouse

150) *What is the name given to a female mouse?*

   a) Boar
   b) Sow
   c) Doe
   d) Buck

151) *Which ONE of the following species does NOT occur as a long-haired variety?*

   a) Mouse
   b) Chinchilla
   c) Hamster
   d) Guinea pig

152) *Which ONE of the following BEST describes the reproductive cycle of the rat?*

   a) Seasonally polyoestrus
   b) Polyoestrus
   c) Monoestrus
   d) Dioestrus

153) *Which ONE of the following species does NOT build a nest in preparation for parturition?*

   a) Mouse
   b) Hamster
   c) Gerbil
   d) Guinea pig

154) *What is the dental formula of the adult mouse?*

   a) 1/1, 0/0, 0/0, 3/3
   b) 1/1, 0/0, 1/1, 3/3
   c) 1/1, 0/0, 2/1, 3/3
   d) 2/1, 0/0, 2/3, 3/3

155) *What is the MOST popular species of gerbil kept as a pet?*

   a) Syrian gerbil
   b) Chinese gerbil
   c) Jird
   d) Mongolian gerbil

156)   *Which species of animal MAY carry out 'foot drumming' behaviour when aroused or aware of danger?*

a) Hamster
b) Guinea pig
c) Gerbil
d) Chinchilla

157)   *Which species of animal would be MOST appropriately housed in a glass tank with a deep substrate of peat and shavings?*

a) Chinchilla
b) Gerbil
c) Guinea pig
d) Mouse

158)   *Which species of animal would you expect to consume the LEAST amount of water per g bodyweight?*

a) Gerbil
b) Rat
c) Mouse
d) Rabbit

159)   *To what order does the chipmunk belong?*

a) Carnivora
b) Rodentia
c) Lagomorpha
d) Mustela

160) *Which ONE of the following species is the act of mating essential for ovulation?*

    a) Rabbit

    b) Mouse

    c) Hamster

    d) Gerbil

161) *In which ONE of the following species is the male referred to as a hob?*

    a) Rat

    b) Ferret

    c) Rabbit

    d) Chinchilla

162) *Which ONE of the following species has NOT been farmed for its fur?*

    a) Chinchilla

    b) Rabbit

    c) Ferret

    d) Guinea pig

163) *Which ONE of the following species can be trained to use a litter tray?*

    a) Mouse

    b) Rat

    c) Ferret

    d) Guinea pig

164) *Which ONE of the following would form the MOST suitable diet for a ferret?*

   a) Tinned dog food
   b) Tinned cat food
   c) Soaked, dried dog food
   d) Any of the above

165) *Which ONE of the following describes the reproductive cycle of the ferret?*

   a) Seasonally polyoestrus
   b) Polyoestrus
   c) Monoestrus
   d) Dioestrus

166) *Which ONE of the following has an os penis?*

   a) Gerbil
   b) Chinchilla
   c) Rabbit
   d) Ferret

167) *Which ONE of the following species is an induced ovulator?*

   a) Chinchilla
   b) Hamster
   c) Ferret
   d) Rat

168) *The female of which species is prone to oestrogen-induced anaemia if left entire in the absence of a male?*

a) Chinchilla
b) Hamster
c) Ferret
d) Rat

169) *Which ONE of the following species should be vaccinated against distemper?*

a) Chinchilla
b) Hamster
c) Ferret
d) Rat

170) *In which of the following species do the testicles descend into the scrotum when the male is 'in season'?*

a) Chinchilla
b) Hamster
c) Ferret
d) Rat

171) *Which species of animal is LIKELY to shed patches of fur if handled in a rough manner?*

a) Chinchilla
b) Hamster
c) Ferret
d) Rat

172) *Which ONE of the following species can be described as monogamous, forming pairs for life?*

a) Gerbil
b) Chinchilla
c) Hamster
d) Rabbit

173) *Which species has a scent gland located along the ventral midline of the abdomen?*

a) Gerbil
b) Chinchilla
c) Hamster
d) Rabbit

174) *Which ONE of the following species is susceptible to 'wet tail' (proliferative ileitis)?*

a) Chinchilla
b) Rat
c) Hamster
d) Mouse

175) *In which species would you administer fluid therapy via the lateral ear vein?*

a) Chinchilla
b) Rabbit
c) Guinea pig
d) Rat

176) *Which ONE of the following species builds a nest prior to parturition?*

   a) Chinchilla
   b) Rabbit
   c) Guinea pig
   d) All of the above

177) *Which ONE of the following species is prone to malocclusion?*

   a) Rabbit
   b) Chinchilla
   c) Guinea pig
   d) All of the above

178) *Which species may excrete turbid brown/red urine in the healthy animal?*

   a) Rabbit
   b) Chinchilla
   c) Guinea pig
   d) Gerbil

179) *Which ONE of the following species does NOT exist in the 'Dutch' coat markings?*

   a) Chinchilla
   b) Rabbit
   c) Mouse
   d) Guinea pig

180) *Which ONE of the following species can be described as 'hooded'?*

a) Chinchilla
b) Mouse
c) Rat
d) Guinea pig

181) *Which ONE of the following species has young called kits?*

a) Chinchilla
b) Rabbit
c) Ferret
d) Guinea pig

182) *Which ONE of the following species has young that are able to sample adult food during the first day post partum?*

a) Rabbit
b) Guinea pig
c) Ferret
d) Rat

183) *Which ONE of the following birds can be classified as a passerine?*

a) Canary
b) Budgerigar
c) Cockatiel
d) African grey parrot

184) *Which ONE of the following birds can be classified as a psitticine?*

   a) Canary
   b) Zebra finch
   c) Bengalese finch
   d) Budgerigar

185) *Which ONE of the following BEST describes the beak shape and foot structure of a psittacine?*

   a) Pointed beak with three toes pointing forward and one pointing backwards
   b) Pointed beak with two toes pointing forward and two toes pointing backwards
   c) Hooked beak with three toes pointing forward and one pointing backward
   d) Hooked beak with two toes pointing forwards and two toes pointing backwards

186) *Which ONE of the following species can be described as 'a medium sized grey parrot with a short, red tail'?*

   a) Cockatoo
   b) Cockatiel
   c) Lovebird
   d) African grey

187) *Which ONE of the following species CANNOT be sexed by visual examination alone?*

a) Cockatiel
b) Budgerigar
c) Canary
d) Zebra finch

188) *Which ONE of the following species is the SMALLEST in size, when adult?*

a) Cockatiel
b) Budgerigar
c) Canary
d) Zebra finch

189) *What is the BEST material for perches in a bird cage?*

a) Plastic
b) Metal
c) Wooden dowling
d) Wooden tree branches

190) *Which ONE of the following species can be classified as a soft bill?*

a) African grey parrot
b) Mynah bird
c) Canary
d) Budgerigar

191) *Which ONE of the following species would be preferable to house in an aviary with canaries?*

a) African grey parrot
b) Cockatiel
c) Zebra finch
d) All of the above

192) *What is the correct name for the glandular or acid stomach of the bird?*

a) Ventriculus
b) Crop
c) Proventriculus
d) Aretonotriculus

193) *What is the function of the crop in birds?*

a) Grinds food
b) Storage organ
c) Produces digestive enzymes
d) Has no function

194) *In birds, what is the name given to the MOST distal part of the digestive tract where waste is excreted?*

a) Anus
b) Colon
c) Cloaca
d) Ano-genital orifice

195) *To which order of birds does the budgerigar belong?*

   a) Psittaciformes
   b) Passeriformes
   c) Falconiformes
   d) Stringiformes

196) *In which species is vitamin A deficiency common?*

   a) Budgerigars
   b) Mynah birds
   c) African grey parrots
   d) Cockatiels

197) *In which species is iodine deficiency common?*

   a) Budgerigars
   b) Mynah birds
   c) African grey parrots
   d) Cockatiels

198) *Which ONE of the following clinical signs is common in iodine deficiency?*

   a) Diarrhoea
   b) Respiratory difficulties
   c) Oral abscesses
   d) Vomiting

199) *When sexing a budgerigar, what colour is the male's cere?*
   a) Green
   b) Yellow
   c) Blue
   d) Brown

200) *At what age do budgerigars fledge?*
   a) 5–6 weeks
   b) 8–10 weeks
   c) 10–12 weeks
   d) 12–14 weeks

201) *In birds, what is the name given to the feathers that cover the surface of the body?*
   a) Flight feathers
   b) Down feathers
   c) Contour feathers
   d) Filoplumes

202) *Which Legislative Act states that a bird should be kept in a cage that is sufficient in height, length and breadth to allow the bird to stretch its wings freely?*
   a) The Keeping of Domestic Birds Act 1981
   b) The Domestic Birds Order 1981
   c) The Captive Birds Order 1981
   d) The Wildlife and Countryside Act 1981

203) *Which ONE of the following species of bird produces crop milk to feed its young?*

   a) Canary
   b) Pigeon
   c) Budgerigar
   d) Zebra finch

204) *Which part of the digestive tract contains grit that the bird ingests to assist with grinding food?*

   a) Crop
   b) Proventriculus
   c) Ventriculus (or gizzard)
   d) Small intestine

205) *Which ONE of the following species would you expect to lack a well developed caeca?*

   a) Budgerigar
   b) Canary
   c) Barn owl
   d) African grey parrot

206) *Which ONE of the following structure contributes towards respiration in birds?*

   a) The diaphragm
   b) Air sacs in the bones
   c) Well developed lungs
   d) All of the above

207) *Which ONE of the following species would you expect to regurgitate a pellet of undigested dietary constituents?*

a) Budgerigar
b) Canary
c) Barn owl
d) African grey parrot

208) *The diet of which species may contain sunflower seeds?*

a) Budgerigar
b) Canary
c) Barn owl
d) African grey parrot

209) *The commercial diet of which species would be expected to contain the greatest proportion of millet seed?*

a) Budgerigar
b) Canary
c) Lovebird
d) Zebra finch

210) *The male and female of which species can be differentiated only by listening to its song?*

a) Budgerigar
b) Canary
c) Lovebird
d) Zebra finch

211) *Which ONE of the following species is housed in a loft?*

a) Breeding budgerigar
b) Canary
c) Parrot
d) Racing pigeon

212) *The female of which species has a brown cere?*

a) Budgerigar
b) Canary
c) Lovebird
d) Zebra finch

213) *The male of which species has bright orange 'cheek patches'?*

a) Zebra finch
b) Budgerigar
c) Canary
d) African grey parrot

214) *Which ONE of the following species may die if their dietary intake of iron is excessive?*

a) Budgerigar
b) African grey parrot
c) Canary
d) Mynah bird

215) *Which ONE of the following species is prone to hypovitaminosis A?*

a) Budgerigar
b) African grey parrot
c) Canary
d) Mynah bird

216) *Which ONE of the following species can be fed a colourant in food that causes the colour of the feathers of the bird to change?*

a) Budgerigar
b) African grey parrot
c) Canary
d) Mynah bird

217) *The budgerigar originates from:*

a) America
b) Africa
c) Australia
d) Antigua

218) *Which seed is MOST common in commercially prepared budgie seed mixes?*

a) Sunflower seed
b) Millet seed
c) Canary seed
d) Hemp seed

219) *The barn owl is BEST described as:*

a) Nocturnal
b) Diurnal
c) Crepuscular
d) Biurnal

220) *The kestrel is BEST described as:*

a) Nocturnal
b) Diurnal
c) Crepuscular
d) Biurnal

221) *How many digits does a bird have on its forelimb (wings)?*

a) 1
b) 2
c) 3
d) 4

222) *In wing clipping, which type of feathers are clipped?*

a) Down feathers
b) Filoplumes
c) Flight feathers
d) Contour feathers

223) *In birds, where is the quadrate bone located?*

    a) In the metatarsal region
    b) At the posterior end of the sternum
    c) Between the tibia and fibula
    d) Between the mandible and the skull

224) *The barn owl belongs to which order?*

    a) Psittaciformes
    b) Passeriformes
    c) Falconiformes
    d) Stringiformes

225) *To which bone do the majority of the flight muscles attach?*

    a) Sternum
    b) Quadrate
    c) Scapula
    d) Femur

226) *Which ONE of the following species occurs in a variety known as 'peach-faced'?*

    a) Lovebird
    b) Budgerigar
    c) Zebra finch
    d) Bengalese finch

227) *In the majority of birds, where is the preen gland located?*

   a) Underneath the beak
   b) Underneath the tail
   c) Above the beak
   d) Above the tail

228) *For which ONE of the following species would dandelion leaves be an inappropriate dietary supplement?*

   a) Canary
   b) Barn owl
   c) Budgerigar
   d) Zebra finch

229) *For which ONE of the following species would mealworms be MOST suitable as a part of the diet?*

   a) Budgerigar
   b) Canary
   c) Zebra finch
   d) Mynah bird

230) *Regarding grit in the diet of a bird, which ONE of the following statements is CORRECT?*

   a) Only soluble grit should be available
   b) Only insoluble grit should be available
   c) Both soluble and insoluble grit should be available
   d) Grit is not an essential requirement and is only required when the bird is kept for breeding

231) *Which ONE of the following would be INAPPROPRIATE when attempting to remove a cockatiel from its cage for examination?*

a) All windows should be closed before opening the cage door

b) All cage furniture should be removed before trying to catch the bird

c) A towel can be used to reduce the chance of being bitten

d) Once caught, the bird should be held as tightly as possible to prevent escape

232) *Deficiency of which mineral would be MOST likely to cause the production of soft shelled eggs?*

a) Magnesium

b) Zinc

c) Carbon

d) Calcium

233) *A cage with vertical bars would be MOST suited to:*

a) A cockatiel

b) A canary

c) A budgerigar

d) A lovebird

234) *What is the colour of the wild budgerigar?*

a) Green
b) Yellow
c) Blue
d) Grey

235) *You are presented with a budgerigar that is believed to be 6 weeks old. How do you confirm this?*

a) By the presence of soft, downy feathers
b) By the presence of black horizontal bars on the underside of its tail feathers
c) By the presence of horizontal black bars on the head that come down to just above the cere
d) By the presence of black, horizontal bars on the back of the head

236) *Which ONE of the following species is native to the United Kingdom?*

a) Zebra finch
b) Bengalese finch
c) Goldfinch
d) Canary

237) *Which ONE of the following substrates would be MOST suitable for an outdoor aviary?*

a) Woodshavings
b) Gravel
c) Paving stones
d) b and c

238) *Which ONE of the following species of parrot is usually white with a yellow crest?*

   a) Macaw
   b) Cockatoo
   c) Cockatiel
   d) Amazon

239) *For which ONE of the following species would fruit be unsuitable as part of the diet?*

   a) Kestrel
   b) Budgerigar
   c) Cockatiel
   d) African grey parrot

240) *A client telephones you at the surgery. A small, yellow bird with a hooked beak has landed in their garden. It is MOST likely to be:*

   a) Canary
   b) Budgerigar
   c) Cockatiel
   d) Finch

241) *Which ONE of the following seeds should NOT be included in the diet of a canary?*

   a) Millet seed
   b) Canary seed
   c) Hemp seed
   d) Sunflower seed

242) *Which ONE of the following species should NOT be kept indoors?*

   a) African grey parrot
   b) Cockatiel
   c) Kestrel
   d) Blue/gold macaw

243) *Which ONE of the following species does NOT build a traditional nest from grasses and twigs?*

   a) Canary
   b) Zebra finch
   c) Budgerigar
   d) a and b

244) *What is the term given to the non-nutritive overcoat of the seed that budgerigars do NOT ingest?*

   a) Shell
   b) Case
   c) Capsule
   d) Husk

245) *Brazil nuts would be MOST appropriate in the diet of which species?*

   a) Cockatiel
   b) Lovebird
   c) Macaw
   d) Budgerigar

246) *Which ONE of the following species CANNOT be trained to talk?*
   a) Cockatiel
   b) Budgerigar
   c) Canary
   d) African grey parrot

247) *Which ONE of the following would be the MOST suitable location for a caged bird?*
   a) In the kitchen away from strong sunlight
   b) In the kitchen by a window that gets strong sunlight
   c) In the living room by a window that gets strong sunlight
   d) In the living room away from strong sunlight

248) *Small species of bird should NOT be kept in entire darkness for long periods of time because:*
   a) They may go blind
   b) They need some light to feed at frequent intervals
   c) They will panic and may injure themselves
   d) They will start to moult and lose their feathers

249) *Which ONE of the following species would make the MOST suitable pet for an eight-year-old child?*
   a) Kestrel
   b) African grey parrot
   c) Budgerigar
   d) Macaw

250) *Dead day-old chicks form the usual diet of captive raptors. These should be fed with a dietary supplement containing:*

   a) Iodine
   b) Vitamin C
   c) Zinc
   d) Calcium

251) *In birds, which vitamin is necessary to ensure that dietary calcium can be utilized?*

   a) Vitamin C
   b) Vitamin B_{12}
   c) Vitamin A
   d) Vitamin D_3

252) *Which ONE of the following species is the 'leutino' colour found?*

   a) Cockatiel
   b) Budgerigar
   c) Zebra finch
   d) a and b

253) *Which type of animal is NOT affected by parvovirus?*

   a) Dog
   b) Badger
   c) Rabbit
   d) Fox

254) *Which ONE of the following diseases does NOT emanate from domestic animals?*

   a) Canine distemper in foxes
   b) Feline leukaemia in Scottish wildcats
   c) Paramyxovirus in pigeons
   d) Feline calicivirus in rabbits

255) *Which colour coat should NOT be worn when handling wild birds?*

   a) Green
   b) Blue
   c) Brown
   d) Red

256) *Which ONE of the following diseases is NOT a zoonosis transmitted by wildlife?*

   a) Leptospirosis
   b) Lyme's disease
   c) Ringworm
   d) Distemper

257) *Which ONE of the following wildlife casualties is NOT likely to be a candidate for euthanasia?*

   a) A swan with botulism
   b) A bird that is blind
   c) A swan that loses its leg
   d) A severed vertebral column

258) *The correct rectal temperature of a badger is:*

   a) 27.8–28.5°C
   b) 37.8–38.5°C
   b) 47.8–48.5°C
   c) 57.8–58.5°C

259) *Which ONE of the following is NOT normally used to locate a pulse rate in a wild animal?*

   a) Sublingual artery
   b) Coccygeal artery at the base of the tail
   c) Femoral artery
   d) Brachial artery

260) *What quantity of oral fluids MAY be safely given to a bird at any one time?*

   a) 5 ml/kg
   b) 10 ml/kg
   c) 20 ml/kg
   d) 25 ml/kg

261) *Which ONE of the following species of tick affects the hedgehog?*

   a) Ixodes ricinus
   b) Ctenocephalides nobilis
   c) Ixodes hexagonus
   d) Nosopsyllus fasciatus

262) *Which species of flea is MOST likely to be seen on a rescued wild animal?*

   a) Ctenocephalides felis
   b) Ctenocephalides canis
   c) Linognathus setosus
   d) Spilopsylus cuniculi

263) *Which species of wildlife are MOST commonly affected by Sarcoptes scabiei?*

   a) Foxes
   b) Pigeons
   c) Rats
   d) Badgers

264) *Which piece of legislation enables a sick wild bird to be caught and treated until it is fit for release?*

   a) Wildlife and Countryside Act 1967
   b) Wildlife Rehabilitation Act 1972
   c) Wildlife and Countryside Act 1981
   d) Wildlife Rehabilitation Act 1988

265) *Which ONE of the following birds must be passed on to a licensed person or a veterinary surgeon if sick or injured?*

   a) Wren
   b) Hawk
   c) Blackbird
   d) Sparrow

266) *The Incubation period of viral haemorrhagic disease in rabbits is:*

   a) 1–3 days
   b) 5–7 days
   c) 8–11 days
   d) 12–15 days

267) *Which ONE of the following does NOT belong to the Mustelid family?*

   a) Badger
   b) Common Scoter
   c) Pine Martin
   d) Ferret

268) *What is the gestation period of a badger?*

   a) 4 weeks
   b) 7 weeks
   c) 10 weeks
   d) 16 weeks

269) *The preferred body temperature of an adder is:*

   a) 20°C
   b) 25°C
   c) 30°C
   d) 35°C

270) *Which ONE of the following birds is NOT listed on the Schedule 4 of the Wildlife and Countryside Act 1981?*

a) Bunting
b) Kestrel
c) Shorelark
d) Pochard

271) *Which ONE of the following breeds of duck can be released into the wild?*

a) Carolina Wood Duck
b) Mandarin duck
c) Muscovy duck
d) Ruddy duck

272) *What is the correct temperature of a hedgehog?*

a) 34–37°C
b) 40–43°C
c) 44–47°C
d) 48–51°C

273) *Which ONE of the following species is primarily carnivorous?*

a) Grey squirrel
b) House mouse
c) Wild rat
d) Hedgehog

274) *Which ONE of the following species is NOT native to Britain?*

a) Red squirrel
b) Grey squirrel
c) Red fox
d) Badger

275) *Which ONE of the following species is diurnal?*

a) Sparrow hawk
b) Barn owl
c) Badger
d) Pipestrelle bat

276) *A client telephones you to say that they have found a fledgling at the foot of a tree in their garden. They do not have any cats in the area. Your advice is:*

a) To bring the fledgling to the surgery
b) To feed the fledgling some bread and milk and then put it back where they found it
c) To leave the fledgling alone and monitor its safety
d) To try to put the fledgling back in the tree

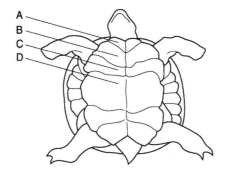

277) *Name the structure labelled A:*

   a) Auxiliary shield
   b) Marginal shield
   c) Insuinal shield
   d) Gular shield

278) *Name the structure labelled B:*

   a) Abdominal shield
   b) Pectoral shield
   c) Humeral shield
   d) Femoral shield

279) *Name the structure labelled C:*

   a) Pectoral shield
   b) Anal shield
   c) Femoral shield
   d) Abdominal shield

280) *Name the structure labelled D:*

   a) Abdominal shield
   b) Humeral shield
   c) Marginal shield
   d) Femoral shield

281) *Which ONE of the following is inappropriate as part of the diet of a Chinchilla?*

   a) Hay
   b) Pellets
   c) Sunflower seeds
   d) Small quantities of carrots

282) *A client telephones you to say that they have found a small squirrel that has stripes on its back with white tips on its tail. The animal is MOST likely to be:*

   a) Fancy rat
   b) Gerbil
   c) Pet mouse
   d) Chipmunk

283) *Which ONE of the following species may start to convulse if stressed (for example if unaccustomed to handling?)*

   a) Gerbil
   b) Rabbit
   c) Mouse
   d) Rat

284) *Which ONE of the following BEST describes the feeding habits of a badger?*

    a) Omnivore

    b) Herbivore

    c) Carnivore

    d) Obligate carnivore

285) *Which ONE of the following is a viral disease that is transmitted by the rabbit flea?*

    a) Viral haemorrhagic disease

    b) Myxomatosis

    c) Toxoplasmosis

    d) Coccidiosis

286) *In which ONE of the following species can the human influenza virus cause death of young animals?*

    a) Rabbit

    b) Guinea pig

    c) Ferret

    d) Chinchilla

287) *Aleutian disease is seen in the ferret. It is caused by:*

    a) Canine distemper virus

    b) A parvovirus

    c) Human influenza virus

    d) Rabies virus

288) *Which type of food is LIKELY to lead to osteodystrophy (soft, deformed bones) in the ferret?*

   a) Tinned cat food
   b) A commercial dried ferret food
   c) Tinned dog food
   d) Raw steak

289) *In which species is the vasectomy of a male appropriate when keeping females required at some point for breeding?*

   a) Rabbit
   b) Guinea pig
   c) Chinchilla
   d) Ferret

290) *Which ONE of the following has the highest metabolic rate?*

   a) Vole
   b) Mouse
   c) Rat
   d) Rabbit

291) *Which ONE of the following is NOT classified as an invertebrate?*

   a) Tarantula
   b) Stick insect
   c) Salamander
   d) Hissing cockroach

292) *Which ONE of the following species does NOT burrow in the wild?*

    a) Guinea pig
    b) Gerbil
    c) Rabbit
    d) Hamster

293) *Which ONE of the following species does NOT practice 'caecotrophy'?*

    a) Rabbit
    b) Hamster
    c) Ferret
    d) Chinchilla

294) *Which ONE of the following species has cheek pouches?*

    a) Rabbit
    b) Hamster
    c) Ferret
    d) Chinchilla

295) *Which ONE of the following species does NOT hibernate?*

    a) Hedgehog
    b) Chinchilla
    c) Hamster
    d) Chipmunk

296) *Which ONE of the following birds does NOT have a crop?*

a) Budgerigar
b) Pigeon
c) Owl
d) Finch

297) *Dimmed, subdued lighting would make all of the following species of bird easier to catch with the exception of the:*

a) African grey parrot
b) Kestrel
c) Budgerigar
d) Barn owl

298) *The diet of a convalescent budgerigar SHOULD include:*

a) A good quality seed
b) Grit
c) Egg-based food
d) All of the above

299) *The name of the fur mite of the rabbit is:*

a) Cheyletiella parasitovorax
b) Psoroptes cuniculi
c) Cheyletiella yasguri
d) Cheyletiella blakei

300) *Which ONE of the following species may exhibit a behaviour known as 'fur chewing' usually in response to a diet low in quality roughage?*

a) Rabbit
b) Chinchilla
c) Guinea pig
d) Hamster

Answers

1)	c	23)	c	45)	b	67)	c
2)	c	24)	c	46)	a	68)	d
3)	b	25)	c	47)	c	69)	c
4)	b	26)	c	48)	c	70)	c
5)	c	27)	c	49)	b	71)	a
6)	c	28)	b	50)	d	72)	b
7)	c	29)	b	51)	b	73)	d
8)	b	30)	a	52)	d	74)	b
9)	b	31)	c	53)	a	75)	d
10)	c	32)	b	54)	a	76)	a
11)	c	33)	d	55)	a	77)	d
12)	d	34)	c	56)	d	78)	b
13)	a	35)	d	57)	a	79)	c
14)	b	36)	c	58)	c	80)	b
15)	d	37)	b	59)	d	81)	d
16)	c	38)	a	60)	c	82)	c
17)	c	39)	d	61)	a	83)	d
18)	b	40)	c	62)	b	84)	c
19)	b	41)	c	63)	c	85)	a
20)	d	42)	b	64)	c	86)	c
21)	c	43)	a	65)	a	87)	d
22)	c	44)	b	66)	b	88)	a

89)	d	125)	a	161)	b	197)	a
90)	c	126)	c	162)	d	198)	a
91)	d	127)	b	163)	c	199)	c
92)	b	128)	d	164)	b	200)	a
93)	d	129)	b	165)	a	201)	c
94)	b	130)	a	166)	d	202)	d
95)	b	131)	d	167)	c	203)	b
96)	c	132)	c	168)	c	204)	c
97)	c	133)	c	169)	c	205)	c
98)	b	134)	a	170)	c	206)	b
99)	c	135)	b	171)	a	207)	c
100)	b	136)	a	172)	a	208)	d
101)	b	137)	a	173)	a	209)	a
102)	b	138)	d	174)	c	210)	b
103)	b	139)	a	175)	b	211)	d
104)	a	140)	b	176)	b	212)	a
105)	d	141)	a	177)	d	213)	a
106)	d	142)	b	178)	a	214)	d
107)	c	143)	c	179)	a	215)	b
108)	c	144)	b	180)	c	216)	c
109)	a	145)	a	181)	c	217)	c
110)	b	146)	d	182)	b	218)	b
111)	c	147)	a	183)	a	219)	a
112)	a	148)	d	184)	d	220)	b
113)	d	149)	a	185)	d	221)	b
114)	d	150)	c	186)	d	222)	c
115)	c	151)	b	187)	c	223)	d
116)	c	152)	b	188)	d	224)	d
117)	c	153)	d	189)	d	225)	a
118)	c	154)	a	190)	b	226)	a
119)	a	155)	d	191)	c	227)	d
120)	a	156)	c	192)	c	228)	b
121)	d	157)	b	193)	b	229)	d
122)	d	158)	a	194)	c	230)	c
123)	a	159)	b	195)	a	231)	d
124)	a	160)	a	196)	c	232)	d

233)	b	250)	d	267)	b	284)	a
234)	a	251)	d	268)	b	285)	b
235)	c	252)	d	269)	c	286)	c
236)	c	253)	c	270)	d	287)	b
237)	d	254)	d	271)	c	288)	d
238)	b	255)	d	272)	a	289)	d
239)	a	256)	d	273)	d	290)	a
240)	b	257)	a	274)	b	291)	c
241)	d	258)	b	275)	a	292)	a
242)	c	259)	a	276)	c	293)	c
243)	c	260)	d	277)	d	294)	b
244)	d	261)	c	278)	c	295)	b
245)	c	262)	d	279)	a	296)	c
246)	c	263)	a	280)	a	297)	d
247)	d	264)	c	281)	c	298)	d
248)	b	265)	b	282)	d	299)	a
249)	c	266)	a	283)	a	300)	b

Printed and bound by CPI Group (UK) Ltd, Croydon, CR0 4YY

03/10/2024

01040848-0006